OSTEOPOROSIS DIET
COOKBOOK FOR VEGANS

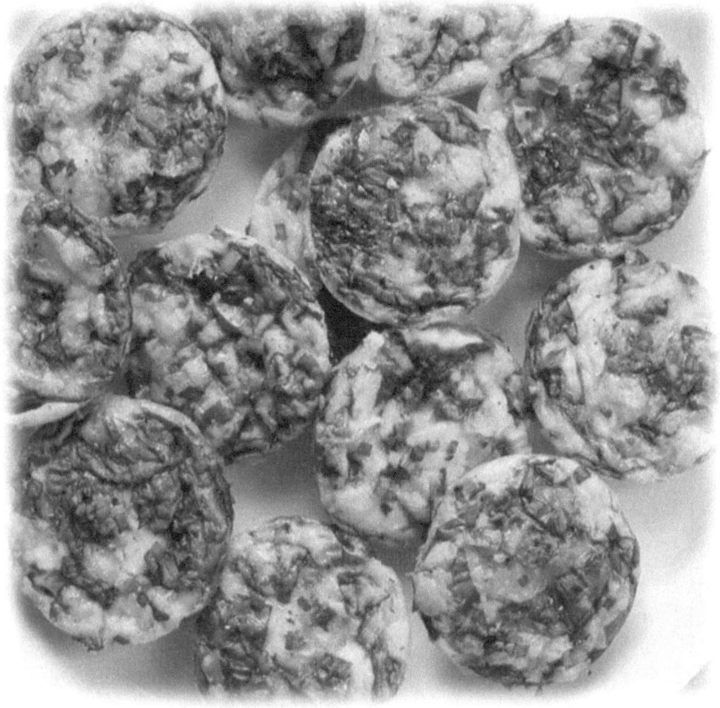

Delicious Plant-Based Recipe to Promote Bone Health

LAKEISHA   OWENS

TABLE OF CONTENT

INTRODUCTION

"Osteoporosis Diet Cookbook for Vegans" readers embark on a transformative journey to navigate the challenges of maintaining bone health while adhering to a vegan lifestyle. Osteoporosis, a condition characterized by weakened bones and an increased risk of fractures, poses a significant health concern worldwide. Traditionally, dietary recommendations for preventing and managing osteoporosis have emphasized nutrients found abundantly in animal products. This book bridges the gap, offering a comprehensive guide that not only demystifies osteoporosis but also presents a plethora of nutritional strategies and delicious recipes tailored for those who choose plant-based diets.

Crafted with the expertise of nutritionists, dietitians, and culinary professionals who specialize in vegan nutrition, this cookbook serves as an indispensable resource for anyone looking to support bone health without compromising their ethical or dietary preferences. It begins with a foundational understanding of osteoporosis, including its causes, risk factors, and the pivotal role of diet in prevention and management.

The book delves into the science of bone health, highlighting essential nutrients such as calcium, vitamin D, magnesium, and protein, and their plant-based sources, ensuring that readers are well-equipped to nourish their bones effectively. The heart of the cookbook features a diverse array of recipes, meticulously designed to incorporate bone-strengthening nutrients into every meal. From vibrant breakfasts and hearty main dishes to nutritious snacks and decadent desserts, each recipe is not only a step towards better bone health but also a celebration of vegan cuisine. The dishes are crafted to be accessible to cooks of all skill levels, with clear instructions and tips for maximizing nutritional benefits.

Moreover, "Osteoporosis Diet Cookbook for Vegans" goes beyond just recipes. It offers practical advice for adapting to a bone-healthy vegan diet in sustainable and enjoyable ways. Whether you are newly diagnosed with osteoporosis, looking to prevent it, or simply seeking to enhance your vegan diet, this book provides the tools and inspiration needed to embark on a journey towards stronger bones and overall well-being.

HAPPY COOKING!!!!!!!!!!!!!!

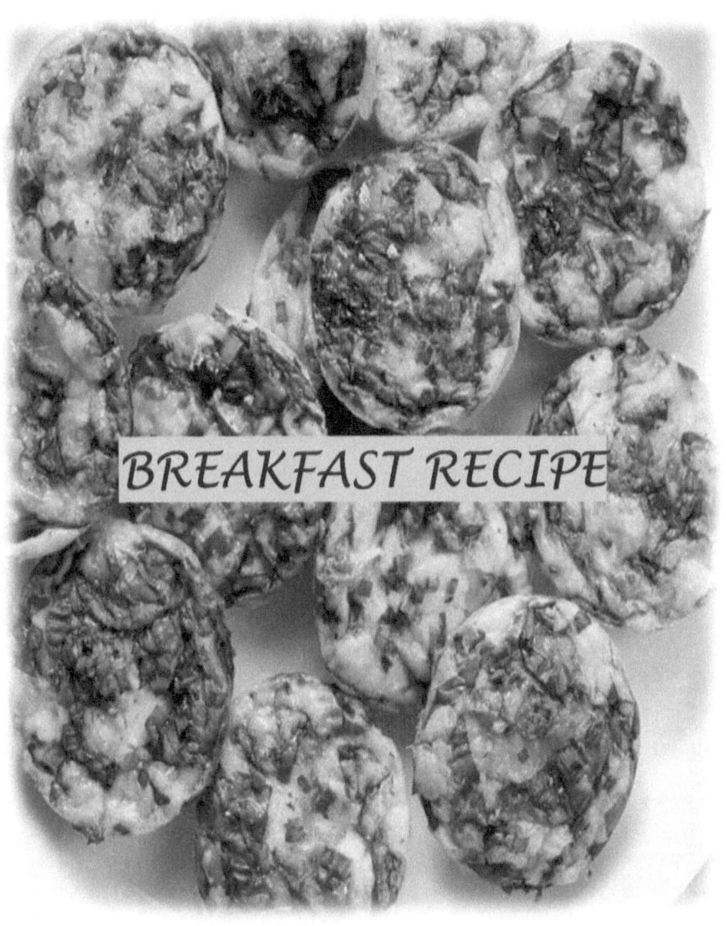
BREAKFAST RECIPE

RECIPE

BREAKFAST RECIPE

Chia Pudding

Ingredients:

3 tablespoons chia seeds

1 cup fortified plant milk (such as almond or soy)

1 tablespoon maple syrup

½ teaspoon vanilla extract, and

A handful of berries.

Instructions:

Mix chia seeds, plant milk, maple syrup, and vanilla in a bowl.

Let it sit overnight in the fridge.

Top with berries before serving.

Tofu Scramble with Spinach and Mushrooms

Ingredients:

200g firm tofu

1 cup spinach

½ cup sliced mushrooms

¼ teaspoon turmeric

Salt, and pepper to taste, and

1 tablespoon olive oil.

Instructions:

Heat oil in a pan, sauté mushrooms until golden

Crumble tofu into the pan, add turmeric, salt, and pepper.

Stir in spinach until wilted.

Almond Butter and Banana Toast on Fortified Bread

Ingredients:

2 slices of fortified whole grain bread

2 tablespoons almond butter

1 sliced banana, and

A sprinkle of chia seeds.

Instructions:

Toast the bread, spread almond butter on each slice.

Top with banana slices.

Sprinkle with chia seeds.

Vegan Yogurt Parfait with Mixed Berries and Nuts

Ingredients:

1 cup vegan yogurt (calcium-fortified if possible)

½ cup mixed berries

¼ cup mixed nuts (almonds, walnuts), and

A drizzle of agave syrup.

Instructions:

Layer yogurt, berries, and nuts in a glass.

Repeat layers and drizzle with agave syrup.

Savory Chickpea Pancakes

Ingredients:

1 cup chickpea flour

1 ¼ cups water

Salt, and pepper

½ cup diced vegetables (bell peppers, onions, spinach)

1 tablespoon olive oil.

Instructions:

Whisk chickpea flour, water, salt, and pepper.

Stir in vegetables.

Cook pancakes in a non-stick pan with olive oil until golden on both sides.

Sweet Potato and Kale Hash

Ingredients:

1 large sweet potato (diced)

1 cup kale (chopped)

½ onion (diced)

2 cloves garlic (minced)

Salt

Pepper, and

2 tablespoons olive oil.

Instructions:

Sauté onion and garlic in oil, add sweet potatoes, cook until tender.

Add kale, season with salt and pepper, and cook until wilted.

Vegan Blueberry and Walnut Oatmeal

Ingredients:

1 cup rolled oats

2 cups fortified plant milk

½ cup blueberries

¼ cup walnuts, and

Maple syrup to taste.

Instructions:

Cook oats in plant milk, stirring occasionally.

Once done, top with blueberries, walnuts, and a drizzle of

maple syrup.

Broccoli and Red Pepper Mini Frittatas

Ingredients:

1 cup chickpea flour

2 cups water

1 cup chopped broccoli

½ cup diced red pepper

Salt, and pepper.

Instructions:

Whisk chickpea flour and water, season with salt and pepper.

Stir in vegetables.

Pour into muffin tins and bake at 375°F (190°C) until set.

Avocado and Spinach Smoothie

Ingredients:

1 ripe avocado

1 cup spinach

1 banana

1 cup fortified plant milk, and

1 tablespoon flaxseeds.

Instructions:

Blend all ingredients until smooth.

Add ice or water to reach desired consistency.

Buckwheat Pancakes with Fruit Compote

Ingredients:

1 cup buckwheat flour

1 ½ cups fortified plant milk

1 tablespoon baking powder

1 tablespoon apple cider vinegar, and

Fruit compote (berries, maple syrup).

Instructions:

Mix buckwheat flour, plant milk, baking powder, and vinegar to form a batter.

Cook pancakes on a non-stick pan.

Serve with warm fruit compote.

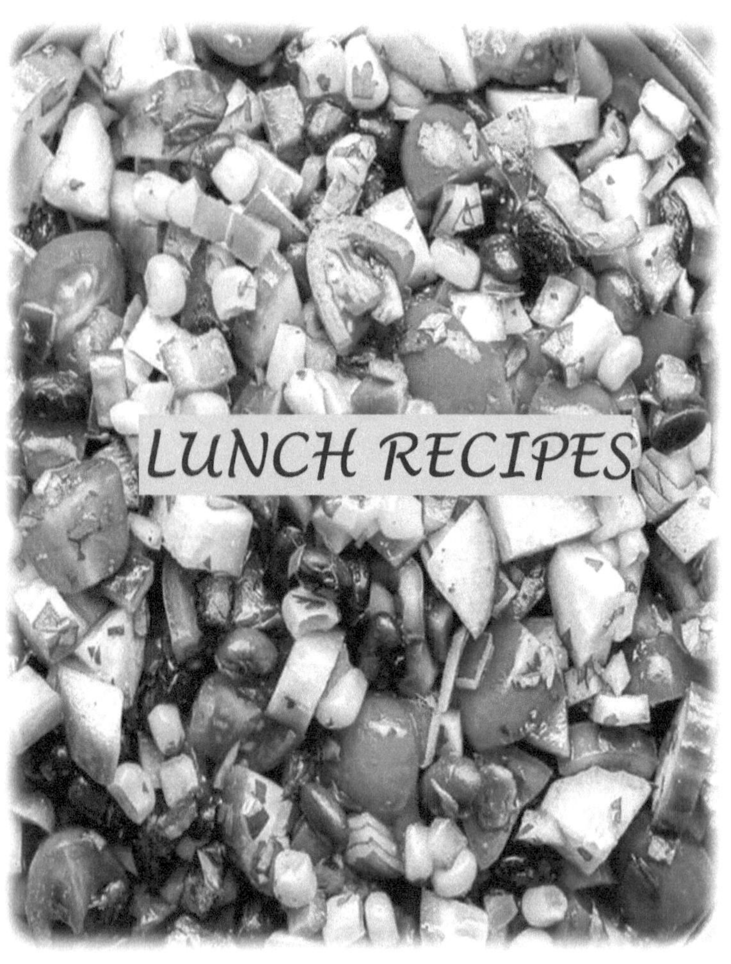
LUNCH RECIPES

LUNCH RECIPES

Kale and Avocado Salad with Almonds

Ingredients:

Kale (chopped) - 2 cups

Avocado (diced) - 1

Sliced almonds - 1/4 cup

Cherry tomatoes (halved) - 1/2 cup

Lemon juice - 2 tablespoons

Olive oil - 1 tablespoon

Salt and pepper to taste

Instructions:

Toss all ingredients in a large bowl.

Season with salt and pepper.

Lentil and Sweet Potato Soup

Ingredients:

Dried lentils - 1 cup

Sweet potato (diced) - 1 medium

Carrot (diced) - 1

Onion (diced) - 1

Vegetable broth - 4 cups

Cumin - 1 teaspoon

Olive oil - 1 tablespoon

Salt and pepper to taste

Instructions:

Sauté onion, carrot, and sweet potato in oil until softened.

Add lentils, broth, and cumin.

Simmer until lentils are tender.

Stuffed Bell Peppers with Black Beans and Corn

Ingredients:

Bell peppers (halved and deseeded) - 4

Black beans (cooked) - 1 cup

Corn kernels - 1 cup

Onion (diced) - 1

Garlic (minced) - 2 cloves

Cumin - 1 teaspoon

Olive oil - 1 tablespoon

Salt and pepper to taste

Instructions:

Sauté onion and garlic.

Mix with beans, corn, and spices.

Stuff peppers.

Bake at 375°F (190°C) until peppers are tender.

Broccoli and Almond Stir-Fry

Ingredients:

Broccoli florets - 2 cups

Sliced almonds - 1/4 cup

Garlic (minced) - 2 cloves

Soy sauce - 2 tablespoons

Sesame oil - 1 tablespoon

Maple syrup - 1 teaspoon

Instructions:

Stir-fry broccoli and garlic in sesame oil.

Add almonds, soy sauce, and maple syrup.

Cook until broccoli is tender but crisp.

Creamy Mushroom and Spinach Pasta

Ingredients:

Whole grain pasta - 8 ounces

Sliced mushrooms - 2 cups

Spinach - 2 cups

Onion (diced) - 1

Garlic (minced) - 2 cloves

Cashews (soaked and blended) - 1/2 cup

Nutritional yeast - 2 tablespoons

Vegetable broth - 1/2 cup

Olive oil - 1 tablespoon

Salt and pepper to taste

Instructions:

Cook pasta.

Sauté onion, garlic, and mushrooms.

Add spinach, blended cashews, nutritional yeast, and broth.

Combine with pasta.

Chickpea Salad Sandwich

Ingredients:

Chickpeas (mashed) - 1 cup

Celery (diced) - 1/4 cup

Onion (diced) - 1/4 cup

Vegan mayo - 2 tablespoons

Dijon mustard - 1 teaspoon

Lemon juice - 1 tablespoon

Salt and pepper to taste

Whole grain bread - 4 slices

Lettuce leaves - 4

Instructions:

Mix chickpeas, celery, onion, mayo, mustard, lemon juice, salt, and pepper.

Serve on bread with lettuce.

Eggplant and Tomato Casserole

Ingredients:

Sliced eggplant - 2 medium

Tomato sauce - 2 cups

Onion (diced) - 1

Garlic (minced) - 2 cloves

Basil - 1 teaspoon

Nutritional yeast - 1/4 cup

Olive oil - 1 tablespoon

Salt and pepper to taste

Instructions:

Layer eggplant, sauce, onion, and garlic in a baking dish.

Top with nutritional yeast.

Bake at 375°F (190°C) until bubbly.

Vegan Cauliflower Tacos

Ingredients:

Cauliflower florets - 2 cups

Chickpea flour - 1/2 cup

Water - 3/4 cup

Paprika - 1 teaspoon

Cumin - 1 teaspoon

Corn tortillas - 8

Avocado, sliced - 1

Cabbage, shredded - 1 cup

Lime juice - 2 tablespoons

Salt and pepper to taste

Instructions:

Dip cauliflower in batter made from chickpea flour, water, paprika, and cumin.

Bake until crispy.

Serve in tortillas with avocado and cabbage.

Sesame Ginger Tofu with Broccoli

Ingredients:

Firm tofu (pressed and cubed) - 14 ounces

Broccoli florets - 2 cups

Soy sauce - 2 tablespoons

Sesame oil - 1 tablespoon

Ginger (minced) - 1 tablespoon

Garlic (minced) - 2 cloves

Maple syrup - 1 teaspoon

Sesame seeds for garnish

Instructions:

Marinate tofu in soy sauce, sesame oil, ginger, garlic, and maple syrup.

Bake tofu until golden.

Sauté broccoli, then mix with tofu.

Garnish with sesame seeds.

Beet and Orange Salad

Ingredients:

Mixed greens - 4 cups

Beets (roasted and sliced) - 2

Orange (segments) - 1

Walnuts (chopped) - 1/4 cup

Balsamic vinegar - 2 tablespoons

Olive oil - 1 tablespoon

Salt and pepper to taste

Instructions:

Combine greens, beets, and orange.

Top with walnuts.

Whisk vinegar, oil, salt, and pepper for dressing.

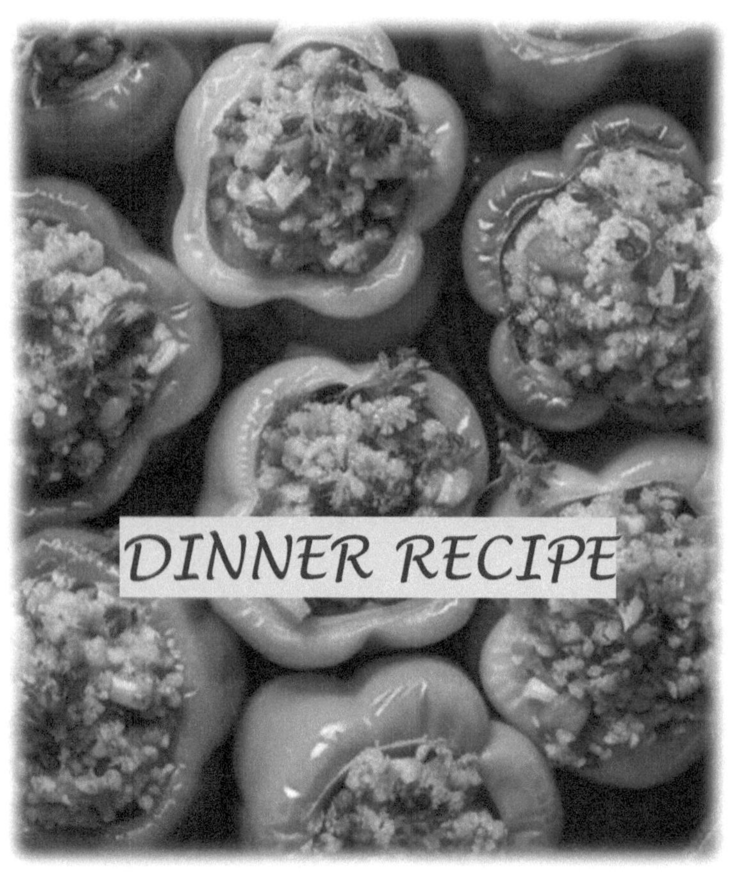
DINNER RECIPE

DINNER RECIPE

Lentil Stuffed Bell Peppers

Ingredients:

4 large bell peppers

1 cup cooked lentils

1 cup diced tomatoes

½ cup chopped onions

2 cloves garlic minced

1 teaspoon cumin

½ teaspoon smoked paprika

2 tablespoons nutritional yeast

Salt and pepper to taste, and

Olive oil.

Instructions:

Preheat the oven to 375°F (190°C).

Cut the tops off the peppers and remove seeds.

Sauté onions and garlic in olive oil until soft.

Add tomatoes, lentils, cumin, paprika, nutritional yeast, salt, and pepper; cook for 5 minutes.

Stuff peppers with the mixture, place in a baking dish, and bake for 25-30 minutes.

Creamy Mushroom and Spinach Pasta

Ingredients:

8 oz whole wheat pasta

2 cups sliced mushrooms

3 cups spinach

1 onion chopped

2 cloves garlic minced

1 cup unsweetened almond milk

2 tablespoons nutritional yeast

1 tablespoon olive oil,

Salt and pepper to taste.

Instructions:

Cook pasta according to package instructions.

Sauté onion and garlic in olive oil until translucent.

Add mushrooms and cook until soft.

Add spinach and cook until wilted.

Pour in almond milk and nutritional yeast; simmer until thickened.

Toss in pasta, season with salt and pepper.

Vegan Shepherd's Pie

Ingredients:

4 cups mashed potatoes

1 cup cooked green lentils

1 cup diced carrots

1 cup peas

1 onion diced

2 cloves garlic minced

1 tablespoon tomato paste

1 teaspoon thyme

1 tablespoon olive oil

Salt and pepper to taste.

Instructions:

Preheat the oven to 400°F (200°C).

Sauté onions and garlic in olive oil.

Add carrots, peas, lentils, tomato paste, thyme, salt, and pepper; cook for 10 minutes.

Spread mixture in a baking dish, top with mashed potatoes.

Bake for 20 minutes.

Balsamic Glazed Tempeh with Steamed Broccoli

Ingredients:

8 oz tempeh sliced

2 cups broccoli florets

¼ cup balsamic vinegar

2 tablespoons soy sauce

1 tablespoon maple syrup

1 clove garlic minced

1 tablespoon olive oil

Salt and pepper to taste.

Instructions:

Steam broccoli until tender.

Mix balsamic vinegar, soy sauce, maple syrup, and garlic for the glaze.

Pan-fry tempeh in olive oil until golden.

Pour glaze over tempeh and reduce until thick.

Serve with broccoli.

Roasted Cauliflower Steaks with Tahini Sauce

Ingredients:

1 large cauliflower cut into steaks

3 tablespoons olive oil

Salt and pepper to taste.

Tahini Sauce:

¼ cup tahini

2 tablespoons lemon juice

1 clove garlic minced

Water to thin, salt to taste.

Instructions:

Preheat oven to 425°F (220°C).

Brush cauliflower steaks with olive oil, season with salt and pepper.

Roast for 25 minutes.

Mix tahini sauce ingredients until smooth.

Drizzle over roasted cauliflower.

Black Bean and Sweet Potato Enchiladas

Ingredients:

2 large sweet potatoes cubed

1 can black beans drained

8 whole wheat tortillas

2 cups enchilada sauce

1 cup chopped onions

1 teaspoon cumin

1 tablespoon olive oil

Salt and pepper to taste

Avocado and

Cilantro for garnish.

Instructions:

Sauté sweet potatoes and onions in olive oil until soft.

Add black beans, cumin, salt, and pepper; cook for 5 minutes.

Fill tortillas with the mixture, roll up, place in a baking dish, cover with enchilada sauce.

Bake at 350°F (175°C) for 20 minutes.

Garnish with avocado and cilantro.

Eggplant Parmesan (Vegan)

Ingredients:

2 large eggplants sliced

2 cups marinara sauce

2 cups breadcrumbs

1 cup nutritional yeast

½ cup unsweetened almond milk

1 tablespoon Italian seasoning

Olive oil for frying

Salt and pepper to taste.

Instructions:

Dip eggplant slices in almond milk, then in a mixture of breadcrumbs, nutritional yeast, Italian seasoning, salt, and pepper.

Fry in olive oil until golden.

Layer in a baking dish with marinara sauce.

Bake at 375°F (190°C) for 20 minutes.

Chickpea and Spinach Stuffed Portobello Mushrooms

Ingredients:

4 large portobello mushrooms

1 can chickpeas drained

2 cups spinach

1 clove garlic minced

2 tablespoons olive oil

1 teaspoon smoked paprika

Salt and pepper to taste.

Instructions:

Preheat the oven to 375°F (190°C).

Sauté garlic in olive oil until fragrant.

Add spinach and cook until wilted.

Mix in chickpeas and smoked paprika; season with salt and pepper.

Remove stems from mushrooms and stuff with the chickpea mixture.

Place on a baking sheet and bake for 20-25 minutes until mushrooms are tender.

Vegan Thai Peanut Sweet Potato Bowls

Ingredients:

2 large sweet potatoes cubed

1 cup cooked brown rice

1 red bell pepper sliced

1 cup shredded purple cabbage

1 carrot julienned

¼ cup chopped peanuts

Peanut Sauce:

¼ cup peanut butter

2 tablespoons soy sauce

1 tablespoon maple syrup

1 tablespoon lime juice

1 clove garlic minced

Water to thin.

Instructions:

Roast sweet potatoes at 425°F (220°C) for 25 minutes or until tender.

Prepare the peanut sauce by whisking together peanut butter, soy sauce, maple syrup, lime juice, garlic, and water until smooth.

Assemble bowls with brown rice, roasted sweet potatoes, bell pepper, cabbage, and carrot.

Drizzle with peanut sauce and sprinkle with chopped peanuts.

Zucchini Noodles with Avocado Pesto

Ingredients:

4 large zucchinis spiralized

1 ripe avocado

1 cup fresh basil leaves

2 cloves garlic

2 tablespoons lemon juice

¼ cup pine nuts

2 tablespoons nutritional yeast

Salt and pepper to taste

Cherry tomatoes for garnish.

Instructions:

For the avocado pesto, blend avocado, basil, garlic, lemon juice, pine nuts, nutritional yeast, salt, and pepper until smooth.

Toss zucchini noodles with the pesto until well coated.

Serve topped with cherry tomatoes.

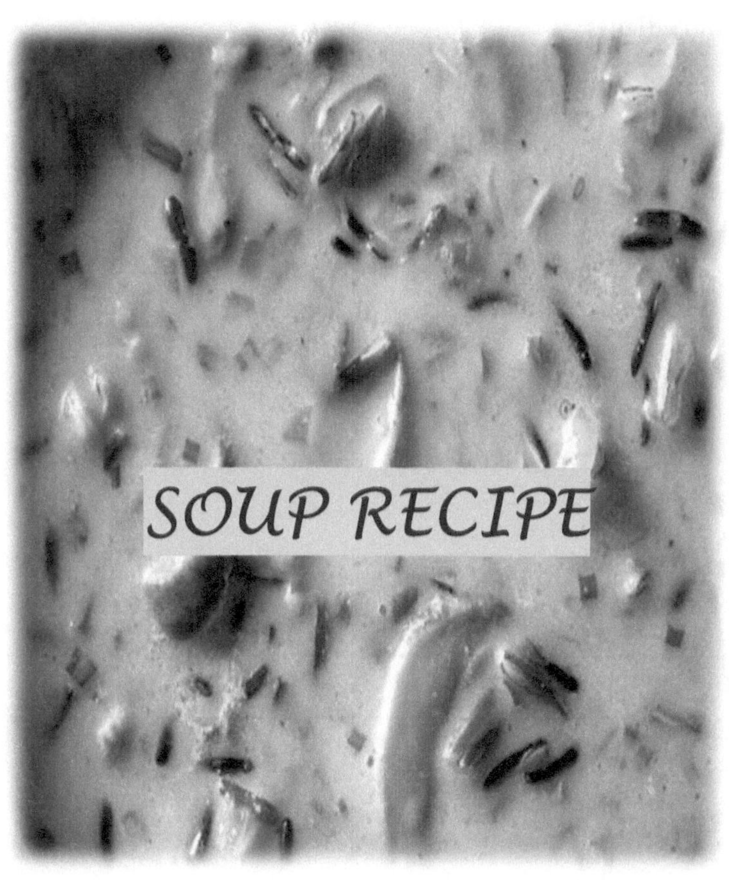
SOUP RECIPE

SOUP RECIPE

Creamy Broccoli Almond Soup

Ingredients:

2 cups broccoli florets

1 diced onion

2 cloves garlic minced

1 cup almond milk

3 cups vegetable broth

¼ cup ground almonds

1 tablespoon olive oil

Salt and pepper to taste.

Instructions:

Sauté onion and garlic in olive oil.

Add broccoli and broth; simmer until tender.

Blend until smooth, stir in almond milk and ground almonds;

season with salt and pepper.

Carrot Ginger Soup

Ingredients:

4 cups chopped carrots

1 diced onion

2 tablespoons grated ginger

4 cups vegetable broth

1 cup coconut milk

1 tablespoon olive oil

Salt and pepper to taste.

Instructions:

Sauté onion and ginger until fragrant.

Add carrots and broth; simmer until carrots are soft.

Blend until smooth, stir in coconut milk; season.

Spicy Tomato and White Bean Soup

Ingredients:

1 can diced tomatoes

1 can white beans drained

1 diced onion

2 cloves garlic minced

1 teaspoon smoked paprika

4 cups vegetable broth

1 tablespoon olive oil

Salt and chili flakes to taste.

Instructions:

Sauté onion and garlic; add paprika, tomatoes, beans, and broth.

Simmer for 20 minutes; season with salt and chili flakes.

Kale and Potato Soup

Ingredients:

2 cups chopped kale

2 diced potatoes

1 diced onion

4 cups vegetable broth

2 cloves garlic minced

1 tablespoon olive oil

Salt and pepper to taste.

Instructions:

Sauté onion and garlic; add potatoes and broth.

Simmer until potatoes are tender.

Add kale, cook until wilted; season.

Butternut Squash and Apple Soup

Ingredients:

4 cups cubed butternut squash

2 diced apples, 1 onion diced

4 cups vegetable broth

1 teaspoon cinnamon

1 cup coconut milk

1 tablespoon olive oil

Salt to taste.

Instructions:

Sauté onion; add squash, apples, cinnamon, and broth.

Simmer until squash is soft.

Blend until smooth, stir in coconut milk; season.

Lentil and Spinach Soup

Ingredients:

1 cup red lentils

3 cups spinach

1 diced carrot

1 diced onion

2 cloves garlic minced

4 cups vegetable broth

1 teaspoon cumin

1 tablespoon olive oil

lemon juice

Salt and pepper to taste.

Instructions:

Sauté onion, garlic, and carrot; add lentils, cumin, and broth.

Simmer until lentils are cooked.

Stir in spinach; season with lemon juice, salt, and pepper.

Mushroom and Barley Soup

Ingredients:

2 cups sliced mushrooms

¾ cup barley

1 diced onion

4 cups vegetable broth

2 cloves garlic minced

1 tablespoon soy sauce

1 tablespoon olive oil

thyme, salt and pepper to taste.

Instructions:

Sauté onion and garlic; add mushrooms and thyme.

Add broth, barley, and soy sauce.

Simmer until barley is tender; season.

Sweet Potato and Black Bean Soup

Ingredients:

2 cups cubed sweet potatoes

1 can black beans drained

1 diced onion

2 cloves garlic minced

4 cups vegetable broth

1 teaspoon chili powder

1 tablespoon olive oil

Salt and cilantro to garnish.

Instructions:

Sauté onion and garlic; add sweet potatoes, beans, chili powder, and broth.

Simmer until potatoes are tender; season, garnish with cilantro.

Cauliflower and Leek Soup

Ingredients:

4 cups chopped cauliflower

1 chopped leek

1 diced onion

4 cups vegetable broth

1 cup almond milk

1 tablespoon olive oil

Nutmeg

Salt and pepper to taste.

Instructions:

Sauté leek, onion until soft.

Add cauliflower, broth; simmer until tender.

Blend until smooth, stir in almond milk, nutmeg; season.

Pea and Mint Soup

Ingredients:

3 cups frozen peas

4 cups vegetable broth

1 diced onion

2 cloves garlic minced

½ cup fresh mint leaves

1 tablespoon olive oil

Salt and pepper to taste.

Instructions:

Sauté onion and garlic; add peas and broth.

Simmer for 10 minutes.

Blend with mint until smooth; season.

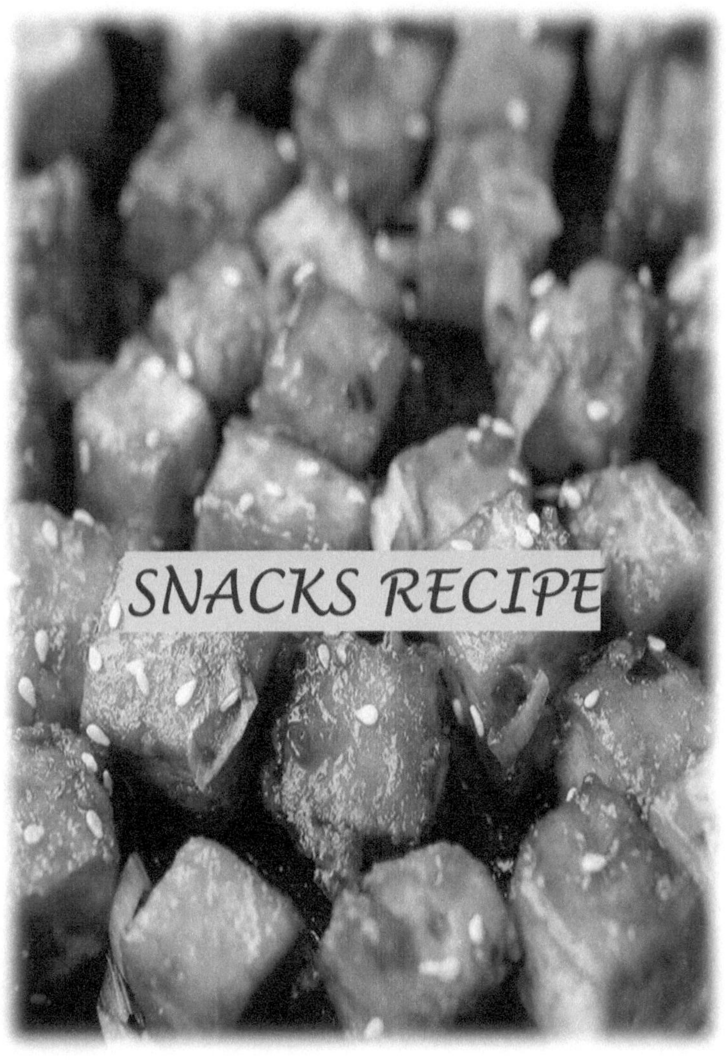

SNACKS RECIPE

SNACKS RECIPE

Kale Chips

Ingredients:

1 bunch kale

1 tablespoon olive oil

salt, and Nutritional yeast.

Instructions:

Tear kale into bite-size pieces

drizzle with olive oil

Sprinkle with salt and nutritional yeast.

Bake at 300°F (150°C) until crisp.

Almond Butter Stuffed Dates

Ingredients:

Medjool dates

Almond butter.

Instructions:

Slice dates open, remove pits, and fill with almond butter.

Roasted Chickpeas

Ingredients:

1 can chickpeas

1 tablespoon olive oil

1 teaspoon smoked paprika, salt.

Instructions:

Rinse chickpeas, dry, toss with olive oil, paprika, and salt.

Bake at 425°F (220°C) until crispy.

Edamame with Sea Salt

Ingredients:

1 cup frozen edamame

Sea salt.

Instructions:

Steam edamame, sprinkle with sea salt.

Carrot and Cucumber Sticks with Hummus

Ingredients:

Carrots

Cucumbers

Hummus.

Instructions:

Cut carrots and cucumbers into sticks, serve with a side of hummus.

Avocado Toast with Hemp Seeds

Ingredients:

Whole grain bread

1 ripe avocado

Hemp seeds

Lemon juice,

Salt.

Instructions:

Toast bread, mash avocado on top

Sprinkle with hemp seeds, lemon juice, and salt.

Baked Sweet Potato Fries

Ingredients:

Sweet potatoes

Olive oil

Paprika

Salt.

Instructions:

Cut sweet potatoes into fries, toss with olive oil, paprika, and salt.

Bake at 425°F (220°C) until crispy.

Vegan Cheese and Apple Slices

Ingredients:

Vegan cheese

Apple.

Instructions:

Slice vegan cheese and apple, serve together.

Rice Cake with Almond Butter and Banana

Ingredients:

Rice cakes

Almond butter

Banana slices.

Instructions:

Spread almond butter on rice cakes, top with banana slices.

Frozen Berry and Coconut Yogurt Bites

Ingredients:

Mixed berries

Vegan coconut yogurt.

Instructions:

Place berries in ice cube trays, fill with coconut yogurt, freeze until set.

CONCLUSION

As we conclude our journey through the "Osteoporosis Diet Cookbook for Vegans," it's important to reflect on the key principles and delicious recipes that have been shared to support bone health. Emphasizing a diet rich in calcium, magnesium, vitamin D, and other bone-supportive nutrients, this book has provided a diverse array of recipes designed to meet the nutritional needs of vegans and those interested in plant-based eating for osteoporosis prevention and management.

From energizing breakfasts and nourishing lunches to satisfying dinners and delightful snacks, each recipe has been crafted with the dual goals of promoting bone health and offering culinary enjoyment. By incorporating a wide range of other nutrient-dense ingredients, we've ensured variety and accessibility in every meal, catering to different tastes and dietary preferences.

It's crucial to remember that managing osteoporosis goes beyond diet alone; it encompasses a holistic approach that includes regular exercise, lifestyle modifications, and, when necessary, medical intervention.

However, the power of a well-planned vegan diet in supporting bone health cannot be understated. Through the recipes and guidance provided in this book, individuals have the tools to make informed choices that contribute to stronger bones and overall well-being.

As you continue on your path, whether you're embracing a vegan lifestyle for the first time or seeking to enhance your existing diet with bone-friendly choices, let this cookbook be your guide and inspiration. The journey to better bone health is not only about the foods you eat but also about enjoying life's flavors and nourishing your body with care.

We hope that the "Osteoporosis Diet Cookbook for Vegans" serves as a valuable resource in your kitchen, helping you to create delicious, nutritious meals that support your health goals. Remember, each meal is a step towards stronger bones and a healthier future.

Here's to your health, happiness, and the joy of vegan cooking!

WEEKLY MEAL PLANNER

WEEKLY PLANNER

WEEK:

MONDAY

TUESDAY

WEDNESDAY

THURSDAY

FRIDAY

SATURDAY

SUNDAY

NOTES

WEEKLY PLANNER

WEEK:

MONDAY

TUESDAY

WEDNESDAY

THURSDAY

FRIDAY

SATURDAY

SUNDAY

NOTES

WEEKLY PLANNER

WEEK:

MONDAY

TUESDAY

WEDNESDAY

THURSDAY

FRIDAY

SATURDAY

SUNDAY

NOTES

WEEKLY PLANNER

WEEK:

MONDAY

TUESDAY

WEDNESDAY

THURSDAY

FRIDAY

SATURDAY

SUNDAY

NOTES

WEEKLY PLANNER

WEEK:

MONDAY

TUESDAY

WEDNESDAY

THURSDAY

FRIDAY

SATURDAY

SUNDAY

NOTES

WEEKLY PLANNER

WEEK:

MONDAY

TUESDAY

WEDNESDAY

THURSDAY

FRIDAY

SATURDAY

SUNDAY

NOTES

WEEKLY PLANNER

WEEK:

MONDAY

TUESDAY

WEDNESDAY

THURSDAY

FRIDAY

SATURDAY

SUNDAY

NOTES

WEEKLY PLANNER

WEEK:

MONDAY

TUESDAY

WEDNESDAY

THURSDAY

FRIDAY

SATURDAY

SUNDAY

NOTES

WEEKLY PLANNER

WEEK:

MONDAY

TUESDAY

WEDNESDAY

THURSDAY

FRIDAY

SATURDAY

SUNDAY

NOTES

WEEKLY PLANNER

WEEK:

MONDAY

TUESDAY

WEDNESDAY

THURSDAY

FRIDAY

SATURDAY

SUNDAY

NOTES

WEEKLY PLANNER

WEEK:

MONDAY

TUESDAY

WEDNESDAY

THURSDAY

FRIDAY

SATURDAY

SUNDAY

NOTES

WEEKLY PLANNER

WEEK:

MONDAY

TUESDAY

WEDNESDAY

THURSDAY

FRIDAY

SATURDAY

SUNDAY

NOTES

WEEKLY PLANNER

WEEK:

MONDAY

TUESDAY

WEDNESDAY

THURSDAY

FRIDAY

SATURDAY

SUNDAY

NOTES

WEEKLY PLANNER

WEEK:

MONDAY

TUESDAY

WEDNESDAY

THURSDAY

FRIDAY

SATURDAY

SUNDAY

NOTES

WEEKLY PLANNER

WEEK:

MONDAY

SUNDAY

TUESDAY

WEDNESDAY

NOTES

THURSDAY

FRIDAY

SATURDAY

WEEKLY PLANNER

WEEK:

MONDAY

TUESDAY

WEDNESDAY

THURSDAY

FRIDAY

SATURDAY

SUNDAY

NOTES

WEEKLY PLANNER

WEEK:

MONDAY

TUESDAY

WEDNESDAY

THURSDAY

FRIDAY

SATURDAY

SUNDAY

NOTES

WEEKLY PLANNER

WEEK:

MONDAY

TUESDAY

WEDNESDAY

THURSDAY

FRIDAY

SATURDAY

SUNDAY

NOTES

WEEKLY PLANNER

WEEK:

MONDAY

TUESDAY

WEDNESDAY

THURSDAY

FRIDAY

SATURDAY

SUNDAY

NOTES

WEEKLY PLANNER

WEEK:

MONDAY

TUESDAY

WEDNESDAY

THURSDAY

FRIDAY

SATURDAY

SUNDAY

NOTES

WEEKLY PLANNER

WEEK:

MONDAY

TUESDAY

WEDNESDAY

THURSDAY

FRIDAY

SATURDAY

SUNDAY

NOTES

WEEKLY PLANNER

WEEK :

MONDAY

TUESDAY

WEDNESDAY

THURSDAY

FRIDAY

SATURDAY

SUNDAY

NOTES

WEEKLY PLANNER

WEEK:

MONDAY

TUESDAY

WEDNESDAY

THURSDAY

FRIDAY

SATURDAY

SUNDAY

NOTES

WEEKLY PLANNER

WEEK:

MONDAY

TUESDAY

WEDNESDAY

THURSDAY

FRIDAY

SATURDAY

SUNDAY

NOTES

WEEKLY PLANNER

WEEK:

MONDAY

TUESDAY

WEDNESDAY

THURSDAY

FRIDAY

SATURDAY

SUNDAY

NOTES

WEEKLY PLANNER

WEEK:

MONDAY

TUESDAY

WEDNESDAY

THURSDAY

FRIDAY

SATURDAY

SUNDAY

NOTES

WEEKLY PLANNER

WEEK:

MONDAY

TUESDAY

WEDNESDAY

THURSDAY

FRIDAY

SATURDAY

SUNDAY

NOTES

WEEKLY PLANNER

WEEK:

MONDAY

TUESDAY

WEDNESDAY

THURSDAY

FRIDAY

SATURDAY

SUNDAY

NOTES

WEEKLY PLANNER

WEEK:

MONDAY

TUESDAY

WEDNESDAY

THURSDAY

FRIDAY

SATURDAY

SUNDAY

NOTES

WEEKLY PLANNER

WEEK:

MONDAY

TUESDAY

WEDNESDAY

THURSDAY

FRIDAY

SATURDAY

SUNDAY

NOTES

WEEKLY PLANNER

WEEK:

MONDAY

TUESDAY

WEDNESDAY

THURSDAY

FRIDAY

SATURDAY

SUNDAY

NOTES

WEEKLY PLANNER

WEEK:

MONDAY

TUESDAY

WEDNESDAY

THURSDAY

FRIDAY

SATURDAY

SUNDAY

NOTES